Travel Survival Secrets

How to Arrive At Your Destination In The BEST Shape Possible!

Angel Tortoriello-Umbach

as seen on:

WBRE

★KLST.
YOUR FIRST CHOICE FOR NEWS

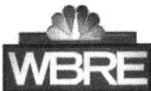

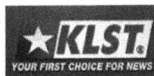

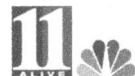

11 ALIVE
A TEGNA Company

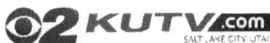

②2 KUTV.com
SALT LAKE CITY UTAH

ISBN-13: 978-0-9908476-1-8
Published by WellYOUniversity Publications
www.WellYOUniversity.com

i

Travel Survival Secrets: How To Arrive At Your Destination In The BEST Shape Possible!

by Angel Tortoriello-Umbach

The author & publisher of this book do not dispense medical advice nor prescribe the use of this material as a form of treatment. The author & publisher are not engaged in rendering psychological, medical, or other professional services.

Disclaimer: The purpose of this material is educational only. Please see you doctor before starting any exercise program or concerning any medical advice you may need.

Travel Survival Secrets

About The Author

Angel is one of America's top
Muscular System Specialists.

She is a nationally recognized expert
and has been featured on
TV networks across the country.

Some of her clients include:

Corky Ballas and Louis Van Amstel
from 'Dancing with the Stars'
and Prima ballerina, Susan Jaffe.

Angel has worked with many
professional dancers, athletes,
children and adults of all ages.

Angel is a certified member of the following organizations:

American Council of Exercise

Resistance Training Specialist

Muscle Activation Specialist

IDEA Elite Personal Trainer

Introduction

In my **years** of *traveling* for

business & pleasure,

I thought about the

mistakes that we can all make.

There were times I would *rush* when

carrying my luggage.

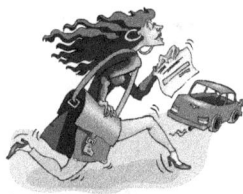

I'd over pack my tote and

sling it over my one shoulder, resulting

in neck & back pain for days!

As I started traveling & sharing

these **very secrets** on

networks across the country –

it occurred to me there was a

better way to share them –

put them in to a book!

So, you are holding **THAT BOOK!**

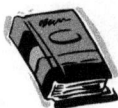

The chapters will take you through

the key areas to watch out for.

Feel free to skip ahead if you see a chapter that you are struggling with.

This book's designed using
SMARTheory -

So it's like none you've seen before!

Not only does it make for a quick read,

information *sticks better* in your brain!

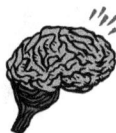

By following the travel survival secrets

laid out in this book – you ensure that you

arrive at your destination in the

BEST shape possible!

Luggage

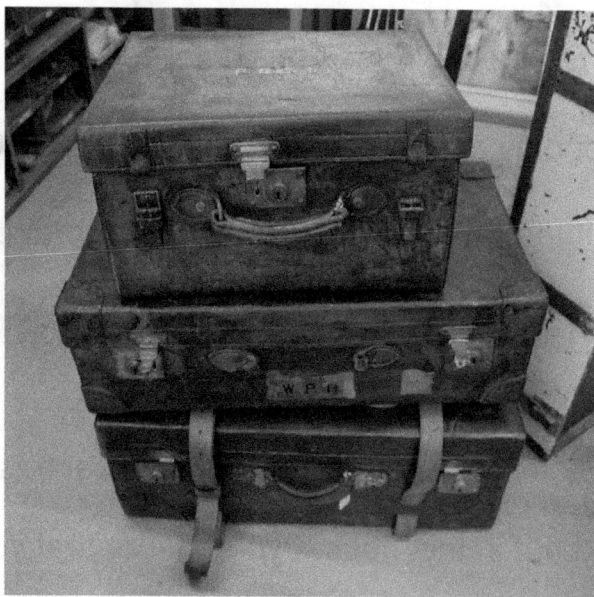

Why It Matters!

53,790

According to:

US Consumer Product Safety

Commission

This is the number of luggage-related

injuries last year!

MOST could have been **avoided!**

To ensure that you arrive at your

destination free from pain -

Follow these secrets....

Survival Secret #1

When **buying** new luggage,

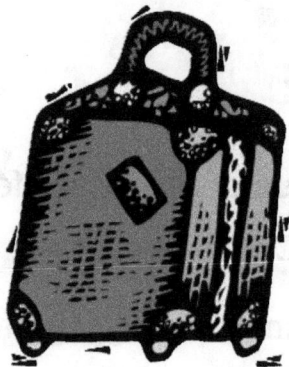

look for a sturdy,

light piece

with wheels and a handle.

Survival Secret #2

When lifting luggage onto a platform
or into a car trunk,

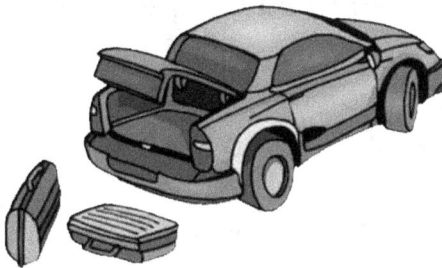

Stand alongside of it, bend at your knees,

NOT at your waist,

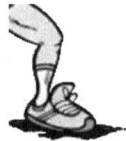

lift with your leg muscles then
grasp the handle & straighten up.

Hold it close to your body!

Survival Secret #3

When placing luggage
in an overhead compartment,

1st LIFT it onto the top of the seat,

place your hands on

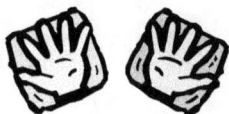

the left & right sides of the suitcase –

THEN **lift it up.**

(or ask a kind passenger to help!)

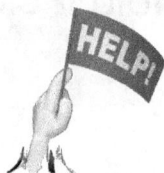

Survival Secret #4

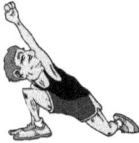 ***DO NOT***

twist your body when lifting

and carrying luggage.

Survival Secret #5

DO NOT

rush

when lifting or carrying a suitcase.

Survival Secret #6

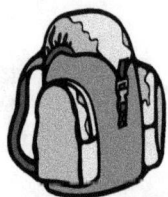

If using a backpack,

make sure it has

padded and adjustable straps.

Survival Secret #7

Don't sling the backpack over one

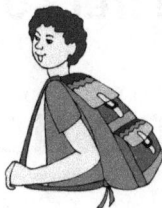

shoulder.

This will cause muscle

imbalance and strain.

Sanitizing

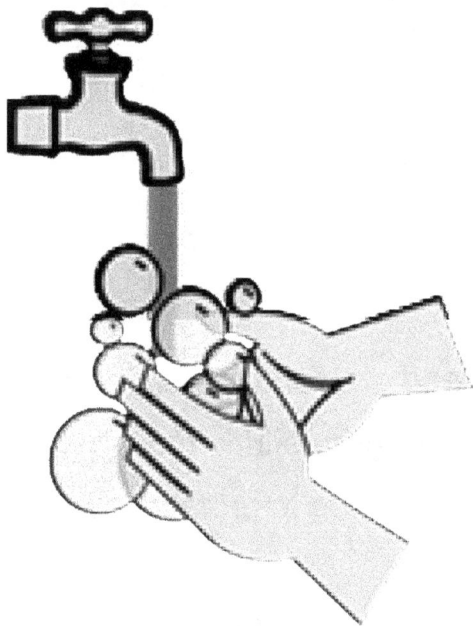

Why It Matters!

Research has found:

People consistently report ⬆ rates of

colds after plane travel with

3% - 29%

complaining of symptoms a week after

a two and a half hour flight or more.

Instead of spending 🕐 worrying

whether germs lurk in every corner,

take steps to protect yourself.

Here are a few tips to arm yourself

against cold and flu viruses.

Survival Secret #7

Pack sanitizing wipes.

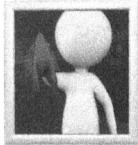

Clean your:

Seatbelt latch, arm rests, seat back,

TV tray table & seat pocket.

Survival Secret #8

Germs like dry air,

so use a saline nasal solution

to keep your nasal passages moist,

which effectively **boosts your body's**

own germ-flushing action.

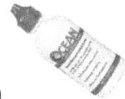

Survival Secret #9

Travel with a face mask!

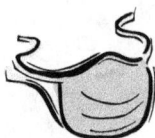

You may never know IF

a fellow passenger is sick.

Survival Secret #10

You might be tempted to close

that air vent blasting
a cold breeze –

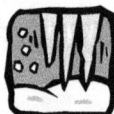

DON'T!

The lack of circulating ventilation

is one of the main reasons

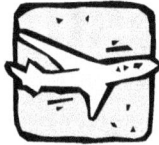

are safe havens for germs.

Actively recirculated

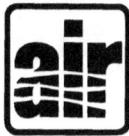

 is filtered -

planes with good ventilation systems

have ⬇

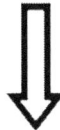

cold & flu transmission.

Posture

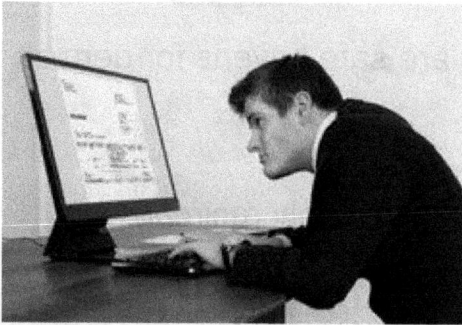

Why It Matters!

Sitting posture affects the spine

The amount of pressure in

the disc is affected by the

manner in which one sits!

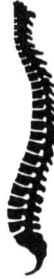

Slouching posture will **increase**

disc pressure & impact the

health of your back

There is **40% MORE**

disc pressure in a *poor sitting posture*
compared with standing.

40% MORE

sitting this way!

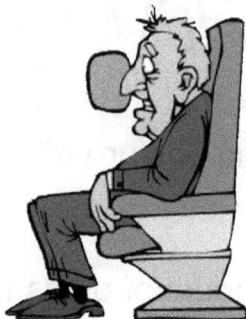

AND

There is an ⬆ of **85%**

DISC PRESSURE when

leaning forward in a poor sitting posture!

Remember.......

Slouching posture will increase

disc pressure & impact the

health of your back.

When the extra pressure is loaded on

OUR DISCS by poor sitting posture -

What can happen as a result is........

- dramatic **increase** in
the ligament force.

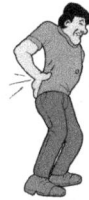

- potential damage to the ligaments
& the disc of the lower back.

Also,

When you sit for a long time not moving,

you lose fluid in the disc.

THIS IS NOT GOOD for your back....

What can happen as a result:

- Disc nutrition gets compromised,

- Lose shock absorbing capacity

- The loss of disc height which ⬆
  the potential for a *pinched nerve*.

WATCH OUT FOR TECH NECK!!

#1) At *15 degrees* of cervical flexion
{looking at your cell phone!}

= the weight of 3 gallons

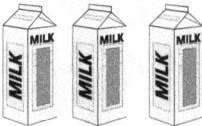

on your spine.

#2) At *30 degrees* of cervical flexion
{looking at your IPAD!}

= the weight of a 5 gallon -
drum of water

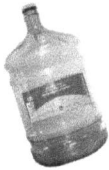

on your spine.

#3) At *45 degrees* of cervical flexion
{reading a book on a plane}

= the weight of 2 tires

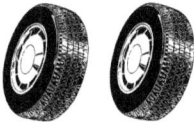

on your spine

Survival Secret #11

Set an alert on your 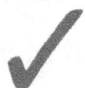 every **50**

minutes to remind yourself to

✓ your posture

&

get up to move!

Survival Secret #12

If you use a tablet or IPad,

invest in a holder that *can attach*

to the **back of the tray table**

(PS. it also works great in the backseat

of your car for the children)

Survival Secret #13

When using a laptop on the plane,

use a portable laptop table

so you are not *sacrificing*

your posture while typing!

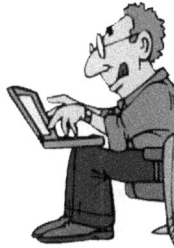

Survival Secret #14

One way to remind yourself about

your posture,

look around & observe your fellow

passengers bent over in their seats!

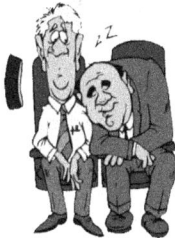

Movement/Exercises

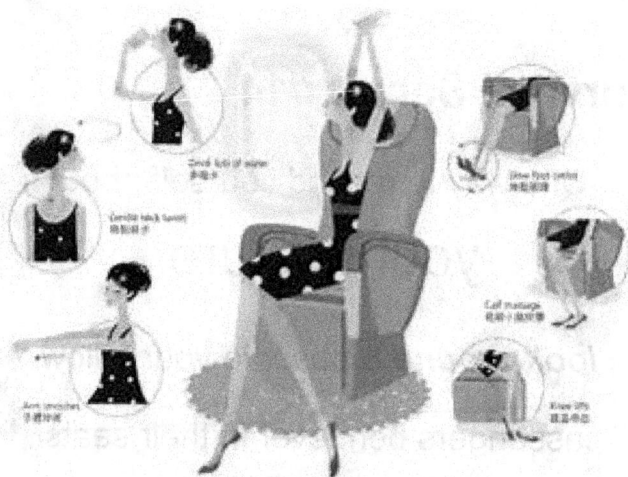

Why It Matters!

The spine is *designed* to move!

Sitting in one position

for extended periods of time

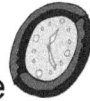

stiffens the back muscles which

can put **stress on the spine**.

Get up & move around every

30 minutes!

Movement

IS GOOD for your back!

There are many benefits including:

1) It stimulates blood flow -

2) Brings nutrients & oxygen to the structures of our back

3) Helps prevent soft tissues in the back from stiffening and aching

MOST IMPORTANTLY

4) **Helps prevent blood clots**

from forming in the legs,

This is called deep
vein thrombosis (DVT)

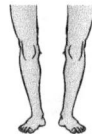

To get moving ,,,,,,

Do the exercises on the next page!

Sitting exercises:

Survival Secret #15

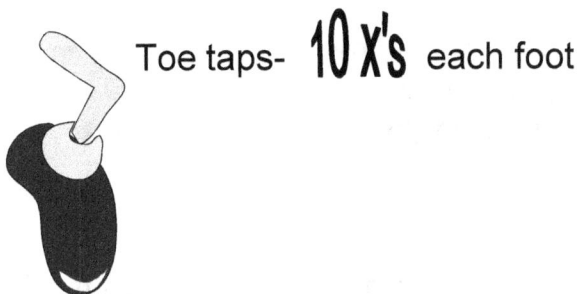

Toe taps- **10 X's** each foot

Survival Secret #16

Heel digs- **10 X's** each foot

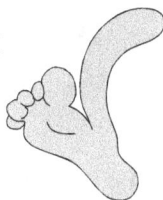

Survival Secret #17

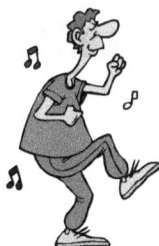

March in place **10 X's**

Survival Secret #18

Triceps pushups –

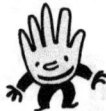

1) Place your palms on sanitized arm rests

2) Straighten your arms

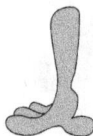

**your bottom should come up from
your seat a few inches

DO 5 to 10 times!

Survival Secret #19

Back exercise - (Lats)

1) Sit up tall,

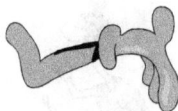

2) Bend your elbows in an L shape,

3) Look straight ahead & **PULL**

   your elbows back toward

   the back of your seat

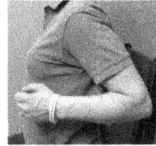

4) Squeeze your shoulder blades

   together – DO 10 times!

Standing exercises:

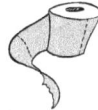

(While waiting for the bathroom!)

Survival Secret #20

   Calf raises

DO 10 times!

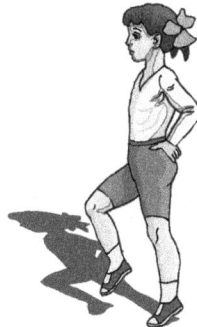

Survival Secret #22

Glute squeezes -

DO 10 times!

Survival Secret #23

Repeat back exercise –

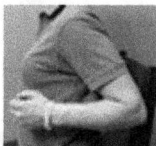

1) Lifting your rib cage,

2) Looking **straight ahead,**

3) Now bring your elbows back,

4) Squeeze your shoulder blades

together – **DO 10 times!**

Survival Secret #24

Potty squats-

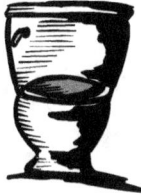

The Key:

- ☐ keep your chest lifted,

- ☐ legs wide, with toes pointing,

- ☐ start to sit deep toward the toilet

AND

BEFORE your bottom

touches the seat,

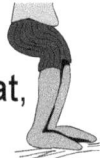

come back up to standing

DO 10 times!

ATTENTION TALL PEOPLE!!

If you are too tall to try this

in the airplane bathroom,

AND

don't mind the looks you may get,

then do the *potty squats*

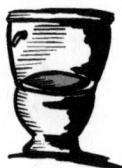

in the **FOOD AREA**

outside the bathrooms!

Food

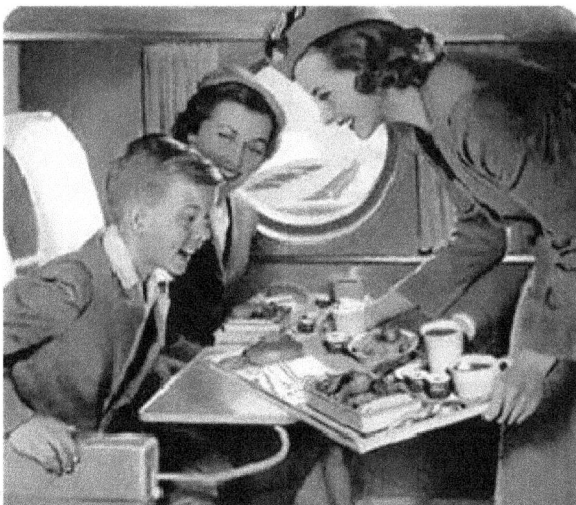

Why It Matters!

If you've traveled by air

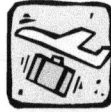

during the last few years,

you probably know that

food options are becoming

more limited on domestic flights.

Some airlines don't offer food at all.

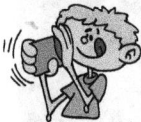

Your best bet if you want to

save **money** &

eat *the foods* you like,

is to plan ahead &

prepare your own meals and snacks.

What To Pack

Here are some of my favorites:

- Dried fruit

- Fresh fruit

- Cheese sticks or other cheese

- nuts(careful of neighboring passenger allergies)

- sandwiches

- raw veggies

- Yogurt / yogurt tubes

- Bagel/cream cheese

- Hard boiled eggs

- Banana bread

- Peanut butter & apple slices

Hydration

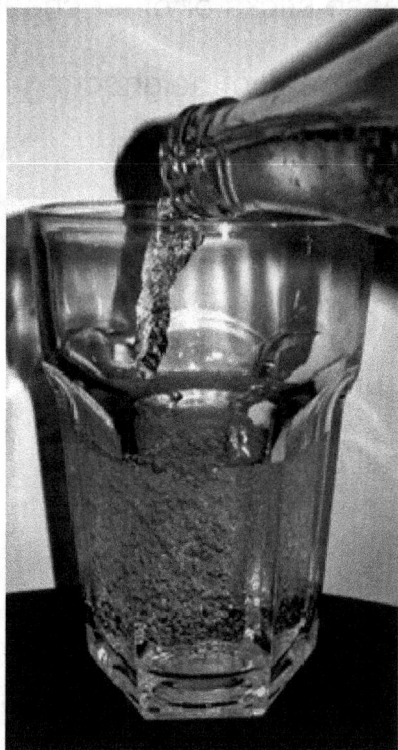

Why It Matters!

Dehydration is a common problem

for passengers when flying,

due to the LACK of humidity

in the air within the plane.

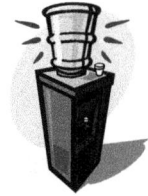

Besides the *uncomfortable,*

thirsty feeling dehydration brings,

it can ⬆ your feeling of travel FATIGUE

& your risk of catching a cold.

Survival Secret #25

Drink **8 ounces** of water

before the flight, and

EVERY hour during the flight

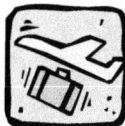

Survival Secret #26

Avoid alcoholic beverages –

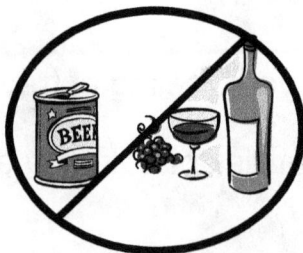

They promote *dehydration*......

Survival Secret #27

Apply moisturizer during the flight

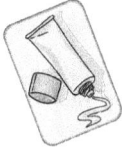 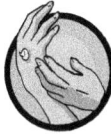

Survival Secret #28

Dab a bit of Vaseline

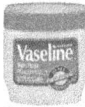

in your nostrils to **protect**

the mucous membranes of your nose.

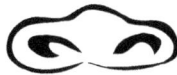

Easy Pack
Check Lists

The following pages were designed to
make your next trip super simple!

Use the following **checklists** to help

make sure you have everything you

need to get to your destination

in the **best** possible shape!

There is a check list for each are!

Rip them out of the book &

USE them as you start your packing!

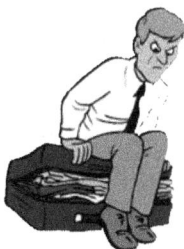

Pre-Trip Check…

☐ Passport or ID

☐ House keys

☐ Airplane tickets

☐ Empty water bottle

☐ Insulated food bag

☐ Saline for nose

☐ Vaseline for nose

☐ Moisturizing cream

☐ Laptop portable table

☐ IPad/Tablet tray table holder

☐ Sanitizing wipes

Food Trip Check.....

- ☐ Dried Fruit/Fresh Fruit

- ☐ Cheese sticks

- ☐ Nuts

- ☐ Raw veggies

- ☐ Sandwiches

- ☐ Hard Boiled eggs

- ☐ Oatmeal cookies

- ☐ Peanut butter with apple slices

Exercise Trip Check....

Seated

- ☐ Toe Taps: 10 times each foot

- ☐ Heel digs: 10 times each foot

- ☐ March in place: 10 times

- ☐ Triceps Pushups: 5 to 10 times

- ☐ Back exercise: 10 times

Standing exercises:

- ☐ Calf raises: 10 times

- ☐ Glute squeezes: 10 times

- ☐ Back exercise: 10 times

- ☐ Potty Squats: 10 times

Pre-Trip Check...

- ☐ Passport or ID

- ☐ House keys

- ☐ Airplane tickets

- ☐ Empty water bottle

- ☐ Insulated food bag

- ☐ Saline for nose

- ☐ Vaseline for nose

- ☐ Moisturizing cream

- ☐ Laptop portable table

- ☐ IPad/Tablet tray table holder

- ☐ Sanitizing wipes

Food Trip Check.....

- ☐ Dried Fruit/Fresh Fruit
- ☐ Cheese sticks
- ☐ Nuts
- ☐ Raw veggies
- ☐ Sandwiches
- ☐ Hard Boiled eggs
- ☐ Oatmeal cookies
- ☐ Peanut butter with apple slices

Exercise Trip Check....

Seated

☐ Toe Taps: 10 times each foot

☐ Heel digs: 10 times each foot

☐ March in place: 10 times

☐ Triceps Pushups: 5 to 10 times

☐ Back exercise: 10 times

Standing exercises:

☐ Calf raises: 10 times

☐ Glute squeezes: 10 times

☐ Back exercise: 10 times

☐ Potty Squats: 10 times

Pre-Trip Check...

☐ Passport or ID

☐ House keys

☐ Airplane tickets

☐ Empty water bottle

☐ Insulated food bag

☐ Saline for nose

☐ Vaseline for nose

☐ Moisturizing cream

☐ Laptop portable table

☐ IPad/Tablet tray table holder

☐ Sanitizing wipes

Food Trip Check.....

- ☐ Dried Fruit/Fresh Fruit

- ☐ Cheese sticks

- ☐ Nuts

- ☐ Raw veggies

- ☐ Sandwiches

- ☐ Hard Boiled eggs

- ☐ Oatmeal cookies

- ☐ Peanut butter with apple slices

Exercise Trip Check....

Seated

- ☐ Toe Taps: 10 times each foot
- ☐ Heel digs: 10 times each foot
- ☐ March in place: 10 times
- ☐ Triceps Pushups: 5 to 10 times
- ☐ Back exercise: 10 times

Standing exercises:

- ☐ Calf raises: 10 times
- ☐ Glute squeezes: 10 times
- ☐ Back exercise: 10 times
- ☐ Potty Squats: 10 times

Pre-Trip Check…

- ☐ Passport or ID
- ☐ House keys
- ☐ Airplane tickets
- ☐ Empty water bottle
- ☐ Insulated food bag
- ☐ Saline for nose
- ☐ Vaseline for nose
- ☐ Moisturizing cream
- ☐ Laptop portable table
- ☐ IPad/Tablet tray table holder
- ☐ Sanitizing wipes

Food Trip Check.....

- ☐ Dried Fruit/Fresh Fruit

- ☐ Cheese sticks

- ☐ Nuts

- ☐ Raw veggies

- ☐ Sandwiches

- ☐ Hard Boiled eggs

- ☐ Oatmeal cookies

- ☐ Peanut butter with apple slices

Exercise Trip Check….

Seated

☐ Toe Taps: 10 times each foot

☐ Heel digs: 10 times each foot

☐ March in place: 10 times

☐ Triceps Pushups: 5 to 10 times

☐ Back exercise: 10 times

Standing exercises:

☐ Calf raises: 10 times

☐ Glute squeezes: 10 times

☐ Back exercise: 10 times

☐ Potty Squats: 10 times

Pre-Trip Check...

- ☐ Passport or ID
- ☐ House keys
- ☐ Airplane tickets
- ☐ Empty water bottle
- ☐ Insulated food bag
- ☐ Saline for nose
- ☐ Vaseline for nose
- ☐ Moisturizing cream
- ☐ Laptop portable table
- ☐ IPad/Tablet tray table holder
- ☐ Sanitizing wipes

Food Trip Check.....

☐ Dried Fruit/Fresh Fruit

☐ Cheese sticks

☐ Nuts

☐ Raw veggies

☐ Sandwiches

☐ Hard Boiled eggs

☐ Oatmeal cookies

☐ Peanut butter with apple slices

Exercise Trip Check....

Seated

- ☐ Toe Taps: 10 times each foot
- ☐ Heel digs: 10 times each foot
- ☐ March in place: 10 times
- ☐ Triceps Pushups: 5 to 10 times
- ☐ Back exercise: 10 times

Standing exercises:

- ☐ Calf raises: 10 times
- ☐ Glute squeezes: 10 times
- ☐ Back exercise: 10 times
- ☐ Potty Squats: 10 times

You can contact Angel -

By phone:

609-439-1861

By email:

Info@MusclesInBalanceLLC.com

Go to:

www.MusclesInBalanceLLC.com

www.ingramcontent.com/pod-product-compliance
Lightning Source LLC
Chambersburg PA
CBHW060637280326
41933CB00012B/2069